<u>FROM FAT TO FIT</u>

This book offers the most practical and amazing way to lose your weight and not losing your hope in achieving one of your important goals of your life of losing weight in very less time of about 4 months or less depending on your dedication and consistency on following the aspects mentioned in the book.

Here you will find all the aspects that are very important and necessary for anyone who is expecting to lose their weight without sacrificing their taste and appetite. You just have to focus on losing weight and follow the steps given and as the steps mentioned are smart steps to lose weight, you will get definite results in a very few months.

The aspects mentioned here are outcome of my personal experiment on losing my weight and I felt that I could have lost my fat more easily and readily if I had them while pursuing the goal of 65kg (143lb) from 90kg (198lb). But now as I know these things I decided to help millions people around the globe to pursue their goal.

There is no ideas or theories in this books and only my personal experience and observation while losing weight and paving path towards fitness. If you follow all the steps mentioned in the book with total dedication and consistency then I'm damn sure that you will lose weight very rapidly and effortlessly.

You will start feeling active and happy from the first week itself of starting to put the aspects into your real life.

Happy Journey FROM FAT TO FIT.

<u>Why this book?</u>

"There are ample of books outside in the market on 'weight loss' so why should I select this book as my guide to weight loss?"

The first reason of choosing this book over other books as your guide is that this book does not contain any fiction, theories or extra and un-important information that just lengthens the book and takes readers much time. So I have kept the data clear and straight to the point helping you lose weight without getting you obsessed to un-important theories and fiction.

Your goal is to lose weight and not your mind so this book is kept as simple as possible so that it can reach to as many as people possible having weight loss as their goal.

Being small yet informative it contains all the necessary aspects you need to consider when opting to lose weight at home on your own without going to gym or other classes on weight loss and spending much of your income.

This book contains basic to advance tips that will boost your confidence and motivate you to start working on yourself right after you complete reading this book.

It gives you freedom to choose your time and place at your home or other place to practice the steps mentioned in the book.

As you don't have to just lose your weight and move on and continue to be healthier, at the end of this book that is after losing your weight you will get three options to choose your path further to a heathier life and according to your dreams and condition you can choose one of them to live the life of your dream.

Fitness is not a destination, it's a way of life.

<u>PREFACE</u>

I transformed myself at the age of 17 knowing that fitness is must to live longer and happier in the 21st century. And it is good to realize this and start working on yourself as early as possible to save yourself from any health related problems. Seeing my huge transformation my friends and relatives were amazed and thought as a miracle has happened to me. Many of my friends and my near ones came to me and asked for advice and tips on losing weight which inspired me share my experience and techniques globally so that all the people wanting to lose weight can have access to this on their desktop or mobile devices. All the techniques mentioned in the book are my own creation and result from self-implementation.

So get ready and be excited to notice the complete process and roadmap FROM FAT TO FAT. Happy reading ahead.

CONTENT

- **ASPECT 1: INSPIRATION AND MOTIVATION**—DISPATCH YOUR MINDSET FROM FAT TERMINAL TOWARDS FIT TERMINAL.

- **ASPECT 2: HABITS**—CHANGE YOUR HABITS SO THAT YOUR HABITS HELP YOU TO CHANGE YOUR LIFE.

- **ASPECT 3: DIET AND NUTRITIONAL INFORMATION**—ALL YOU NEED TO KNOW ABOUT DIET AND NUTRITION TO LOSE WEIGHT. (INCLUDES MYTH BUSTERS)

- **ASPECT 4: PHYSICAL WORKOUTS**— ALL YOU NEED TO KNOW ABOUT PHYSICALLY TRAINING YOUR BODY.

- **ASPECT 5: TRACKING YOR PATH**—KEEPING AN EYE ON YOUR PROGRESSS.

- **ASPECT 6: REWARDIND YOURSELF**—REWARD YOURSELF AFTER ACHIEVING EACH MILESTONE.

- **ASPECT 7: KNOWING A PATH AHEAD AFTER LOSING WEIGHT.**

<u>ASPECT 1: INSPIRATION AND MOTIVATION</u>

DISPATCH YOUR MINDSET FROM FAT TERMINAL TO FIT TERMINAL.

Before you start to implement the steps mentioned in the book it's very for you to get motivated because the start of the journey is little tough and you will require to get a proper momentum right from the start to get to your results as early as you wish. So, I'm sharing below how I got inspired to transform myself from 90 kg to 65 kg.

I was a chubby boy from my childhood itself, yet I started to transform my body when I was 16. Why, was it when I came to know that fitness is must and necessary if you wish to live a long and healthier life? No. I knew it right from the primary school. Then why didn't I transformed myself from then? Because I wasn't inspired by anything or anyone that pushed me to lose weight and step-up towards a healthy life.

But when I was in 10th grade, I was taking coaching from a teacher who was holding doctorate in English literature, who even being above 65 years age was more active and powerful than I had ever met in my life who at this age was this much enthusiastic. He used to travel 12 miles from his home to the center and back without getting tired or did rarely took medical leave, which inspired me and my classmate and so went to him to know his secret.

When I asked him about how did he managed to be such enthusiastic when people of his age had already retired and spending time with their spouse worrying about their health and secure. When we asked him rather he took supplements or vitamins to manage his health to which he laughed and tapped my shoulder in pride and told me that, "Your body is your greatest asset in which you have to start investing right from maturity to get high returns till the end".

I was 90 kg when I asked him this question. He advised me to start losing weight as early as I can so that life can start handing me some of most extraordinary joy, opportunities and freedoms to live an amusing life till end and gave me some tips on losing weight. His lifestyle inspired me to lose weight and start my journey towards a life I always dreamed if I was fit.

The aspects in the book are what he taught me but the way they should be implemented was discovered by me because he taught me to implement them in the old ways-the hard ways. But what I have mentioned here are in the smart ways.

So, now as you are aware of how important it is to have an inspiration or get inspired by something or someone that will boost your confidence and you will get yourself busy in achieving one of life's most important goal of becoming fit.

Becoming fit does not just mean becoming physically fit and having lean body and a trimmed body and a good physique but it also mean becoming mentally fit. And I have also mentioned the workouts for mental fitness in the workout's chapter. So make sure to read each chapter carefully and implement each step with same manner that I have mentioned because it will save much of your time and take you towards FIT terminal in no time and with minor efforts.

Losing your weight will allow you enjoy the most amazing ride in the park near your place and also let you to join any kind of sport you wished to play or make a career in one. Losing your weight will keep you one step ahead of other 31% obese people of the world. Becoming fit will therefore allow you to enjoy the life and your job in your way that these 31% people around world are missing.

You might be seeing your best actor or actress and admiring them for their shape and speech. So just think how people will admire you when you lose weight and went on to become one of the best actors/actress of the world. And for that you just have to take a step of losing your weight.

I know you have got only one life and you want to do whatever your passion is or you love doing or wish being at some position of your dream but cannot do because of your weight so, I especially designed this book in a way that will allow you to lose weight in most effortless way. And your body will thank you for what you did for it.

Now from the next chapter I'm starting the main aspects that will help you lose weight in the easiest way and without giving up your taste. So be excited and fresh to gain all the things you need to know to lighten you.

ASPECT 2: HABITS

CHANGE YOUR HABITS SO THAT YOUR HABTS HELP
YOU TO CHANGE YOUR LIIFE.

Habits are the most important part of your life because your habits itself shows defines your goals and the habits are the only ways to predict your future in any field you are presently working of opting to choose. So in the same way and for the same reason you have to change your FAT habits to FIT habits and in this chapter I will tell you which habits are most important for effective results and forever healthier life and also show the ways to develop them.

I remember when I was in school I used to skip my meals and then having junk food outside with friends. I didn't even paid attention to the meal while having it instead I used to watch T.V. or Netflix while having meals even when I went to hotels I used to eat while seeing Instagram stories or chatting with my friends.

My this habit did not allowed me to have a sense of how much quantity I ate and I always ended having consumed much higher calories than my body actually needed. This on long term increased my weight making me lazy and chubby.

That means, do not have any kind of distractions atleast while having your meals and pay complete attention on your food because chewing your food properly before sending it to your stomach is also very important because if your food starts to digest right from your mouth. So chewing your food properly and nearly 32 times a piece is very good habit.

Doing this you will do most of digesting work by yourself and that will help your stomach to manage the food properly which itself will help your digestive power and improve your health readily without taking anything from you and just by doing it in right way will show you results right from the same day. So from now onwards set aside distractions and keep a count on your calories intake.

Now most of the obese people I see have very bad and common habit of drinking much water just after completing their meal which will no doubt clear your throat and mouth but on contrary it will negatively affect your digestive system and no matter how much you have chewed your food or how much less calories you consumed, drinking much water or any kind of beverages just after your meal will push undigested food in your intestine which will not only create health problems but also you will gain weight.

You can have a sip or two of water just after meal to clean your mouth and esophagus. Even after having couple of sips of water you feel incomplete and thirsty than you can have a half glass of WARM water but never ever have cold water after your meal.

Now second bad habit of many people is staying up till late night with or without any purpose. When you indulge yourself in your office work or any TV show till late night without keeping an eye on the clock then after 2 hours or more then you will feel hungry and you will eat whatever is handy to you. Now after eating you will directly go to sleep without letting your food to digest and so these late night food will directly get converted to fats causing weight gain and even health problems on long term.

If you don't have other option rather than staying up for work then you can have a cup of hot milk with some turmeric powder. This will not only satisfy your stomach but also take care of health as turmeric is a spice that readily work as a medicine. So now onwards if you have to stay till late night then keep a 200 ml cup of hot milk with added turmeric powder handy and your body will thank you on long term.

This habit has helped me a lot to improve my digestive as well as immune system a lot. So make this remedy a habit and you will notice an impressive change in your body and health.

Now, another worse you could have is smoking or drinking just after having your meal. I don't need to explain the worst effects of smoking on your overall body especially your lungs, but smoking just after you had lunch or dinner as it cause a tremendously bad effect on your digestive system as well which will turn your food into fat only causing bad cholesterol in your body.

Also consuming alcohol after meal can lower your liver function and also can cause pancreas not function well, as liver and pancreas plays a vital role in digesting your food and boosts your metabolism will not function well and you will feel lazy and your fat will keep increasing.

So to lose your fat, first you have to quit your habit of smoking and drinking right after the meal. You can have it after 3 hours of having meal but avoid having right after it.

Next very important habit to lose weight and also feel active physically and mentally you have to keep your body moving after each 40-45 minutes to continuous sitting. As you will move your body will have to work and thus the more you move your body will start taking energy from your fat which will readily help you lose fat and ultimately weight.

Along with the above habits there is one more important habit that you should consider to lose fat happily and that habit is- a habit of drinking water after your every short walk of 40 min or more. This will not just help you stay hydrated but it will regularly keep detoxifying your body to bad minerals and fat.

These were some of the major habits that is found very common in many people. So you need to consider each good habit and start

According to me some practical solution on diet that you can follow on your daily basis and as your regular meals. See your main goal is to limit the amount of calories in your diet because ultimately the over-consumption of calories' only results in increasing body fat and thus giving you extra weight. Thus you have to measure your calories intake in your each meal and that should be less than the calories you burn during your workouts. It is my personal experience as I did the same and got results very early and higher than expected.

Some most important nutrition that you diet must contain are, PROTEIN, LOW CARBS, GOOD FATS. Now you might be thinking that as we are here to lose fat why should we consume fat? That's true but here I have mentioned is GOOD FAT and the fat that is stored in your body at present is bad fat which causes weight gain and your weight at present is just due to bad fat.

Some rich sources of protein are whole eggs, seafood, meat and milk. Now the question is that how should they be consumed and at what time?

So, the eggs should be consumed with running yolk and the best time to consume them is in the breakfast along with some nuts. And that is because nuts are rich source or good fats and fiber while eggs are rich source of protein. Never commit a mistake by consuming milk in you breakfast as it takes time to digest and so it will negatively affect your body. Your breakfast can also contain boiled oatmeal with some healthy spices and nuts. That is what I used to have when transforming myself.

But do not consume the food till your satisfaction rather keep yourself dis-satisfied because that feeling to dis-satisfaction will energies you and that will the sign that you have consumed less calories than that you have burned. So never get yourself fulfilled in any of your meal. There are also many other breakfast options that you can yourself create by looking around yourself and measuring the calories intake. In short your breakfast must be the largest and healthiest meal of your day because if you win the morning, you win the day.

Never forget to drink plenty of water during your day as it will not just keep you hydrated but also will it keep your food moving and stop your food from getting converted to fat.

For lunch, you should concentrate on the balanced combination of PROTEINs and CARBs. If you are vegetarian then having whole wheat bread with some fruits and peanut butter is one option. Another option is having Indian chapatti (made from wheat flour) with some green leafy vegetables. If you have high production of rice at your place then you can opt for brown rice along with some curry of vegetables. If you are non-vegetarian then you can go for meat, beef, chicken but remember sharing your food with others as you don't have to consume the whole thing alone as you are watching your calories.

You don't have to rest after lunch as you don't need due to low metabolism but if you cannot resist your sleep then you can just have a short nap during the whole day as you don't have to keep up till late night.

After 3-4 hours of having lunch you can have a cup of black tea, black coffee, green tea or any other drink you like. But remember to have very less or no sugar involved in you drink because sugar is high in calories. But if you have sweet tooth then you can have an apple along with some peanut butter on it instead of having drinks. Or you can go for the chocolate milk but the chocolate should be as dark as possible and milk should be low toned and no sugar must be added to the shake as chocolate itself has some sugar in it. You have got this many tasty snack options so why to go for processed foods like chips!

Till evening you must have to consume atleast 1.5 liters of water. You might have heard someone saying that if you want to lose weight than you have to starve yourself after 6 pm. Caution this is a myth and is totally wrong unless you do not have dinner just before your bed time. I suggest you to have completed your dinner before 2.3-3 hours of going to bed. This is because our food is churned in stomach for nearly 3 hours until then 70% of digestion process is completed and if you don't move your body after dinner and directly go to sleep then your food will not be able to move to intestines after processing in stomach which will turn your food directly into bad fats and cholesterol.

Some foods you should or can consume as your dinner are, if you are vegetarian then you can have light salads of sweet corn, pastas, peanut and onion salad, some fruits along with salads and some healthy and less calories soups minestrone soup, sweetcorn soup, beans soup etc...

For non-vegetarian people you can have sea-food like fish meat, rice with fish curry etc. In definite proportions but avoid heavy foods like chicken meat and beef leave them for the next day lunch.

You might be thinking that I was telling to lose fat while not sacrificing your favorite food. So here it is the way and as per I told you, you can have your favorite junk-food like pizza, burger, fried chips or anything high calories and high starch food of your choice on sundaes. But remember not to have that in all of your meals, you can compromise your one meal but not every meal. I suggest you to have your diet in your breakfast and lunch and go for pizza with coke and ice-cream in dinner.

But remember this scheme is only valid for sundaes and not working days as you have to be highly energized without feeling exhausted at your workouts.

After having known your diet you can set your workouts as per your convenience. But the workouts and intensities you must keep is given in detail in the next chapter.

<u>ASPECT 4: PHYSICAL WORKOUT</u>

ALL YOU NEED TO KNOW ABOUT PHYSICALLY TRAINING YOUR BODY.

After you got knowledge about the diet and nutrition, it is very important to know about workouts and exercises and to achieve your weight goal as early as possible it becomes damn necessary to keep your diet and workout balanced.

You might have heard people saying that to lose weight you have to give up your food and do not bother about physical training or others might be saying that you have to do intense cardio and do not think of balancing your diet. By saying these things, people understands that diet and workouts are two sides of a coin but it's not like that in fact they are two sides of a see-saw, to gain stability i.e. to achieve definite results you have to keep balance on both aspects rather than only one.

Here, I will provide both liberal and intense workouts and trainings to instant weight loss and also some general information on effects of workout on your body and tips and tricks to keep your body on active mode through-out the day even while having intense cardio or full body workouts.

The best combinations of workouts for weight loss is cardio + weight training. That is while having cardio you can do weight training with dumbbells, barbells or just with machines. But, I prefer to use free weights for training rather than going for machines because free weights will not just provide you strength but also develop your physical balance and your mind-body co-ordination will increase as you practice more and more on free weights. I personally used this technique to transform myself. So, it is my personal guarantee that you will get definite results if you follow the technique with consistency and with proper diet.

If you are beginner to weight loss then you should follow the techniques mentioned below.

1. Your cardio must include 10 minutes of jogging either on treadmill or you can go to park. This is the initial stage and at this stage you don't have to start intense but just have to make your body tend to moving and this you have to do for 10-15 days depending on your physical health. If you fell, you have gained energy and stamina for the intense workout then you can start with intense cardio and weight training right after a week.
2. You must feel fresh and active throughout the day and feel more excited than before as this will be the sign that you are on the right track.
3. If you feel tired and lazy in the afternoon after having lunch then it's a sign that your metabolism has improved and so take a short nap of 15 minutes, it will give you energy for the further day. but don't go for a 30-45 minutes rest because that is the time your sleep cycle takes to send you in the deep sleep and so if you wake up after an hour then you might feel more tired and sleepy the whole day ahead. So, avoid a 30 minutes or more sleep rather take short naps on regular intervals.
4. Never go for weight training just after having cardio because as you have given your most in the cardio you might not have further energy for weight training and you might actually ruin your training. So, I suggest going for weight training before having cardio. This is the method I used to follow and this has also helped many people to whom I have advice to follow the method.
5. Do not go for weight training if you are sick or injured because it will make your health even worse and another thing you might possibly not be able to continue for further for a week or more. So, better give your body rest and time to heal. In the mean time you can have short cardio as it will keep you fresh and active and you will fall even during your illness.

Now, if you have gained momentum in your cardio which includes cycling, running, treadmills or anything else you can set high intensities as your body can now bare any kind of push and pull. And some guide for weight training is also mentioned below along with highly intensified workouts.

The best time for intense workouts is in the morning before breakfast because that will directly consume energy from your fat as you don't have any other nutrients present in your body to contribute energy to your body for workout. That is why you can have much faster results if you work-out in morning on an empty stomach. I also did the same and now my body thanks me for the decision I took.

Your intense workout should last no more than 20 minutes as you don't have to take rest between your exercises for more than 30 seconds, that's why it is called an intense workout. There is no secret behind the types of exercises you do but it's the time that you take to complete one exercise. Because once you take rest between your workouts, you will not feel to continue so, it is better not to rest for more than 30 secs.

If you opt to go to gym for your workouts then take someone who has goals same as yours (weight loss), as they will help you stay motivated and you will feel like a competition with them and that will push you to finish your task as fast as possible and that will ultimately help you. But if you choose to stay at home and work-out on your own and alone as I did then set your time goal that will itself compete you to stay ahead of yourself.

Some exotic workouts that I did are 'full body workouts', that focused on my whole body and burning fat from my whole body at the same time so that I don't have spare my time and energy foe particular part of body. And I used to do weight training in the evening as I was unable to manage weight training along with cardio. But always remember to have cardio on an empty stomach.

Along with training and workouts you should also keep moving your body throughout the day. This can be done by dong your laptop work by standing or continuously having small walks of 5-10 mins. At certain time intervals near your office or if you are self-employed and work from your home then you can take short breaks after every hour and have a short walk and a cup of water after walk.

As you do workouts, never forget to rehydrate yourself by having a cup of water after and before workout and also having water after your walks. In short you have to drink atleast 9 cups to water in the whole day without fail.

<u>ASPECT 5: TRAKING YOUR PATH</u>
KEEPING AN EYE ON YOUR PROGRESS

When you go for a marathon or any race, you keep hard on the way to reach the end or finish the race before others to win the race. During that time from begin to end when you get tired and almost lose your hope and immediately you see a sign board indicating just 400 meters to end then at that time you get motivated and regain your hope and successfully finish the marathon.

The same idea or strategy is involved in tracking your progress during weight loss so that you can stay motivated and successfully be able to achieve your goal.

If you opt to go to gym for weight loss and keep a trainer then the trainer will do that do job of tracking your progress. But if you are intending to lose weight at home on your own then it is your duty to track your own progress. I did the same.

The way you can keep a track on your progress is by consciously analyzing yourself during your day and comparing yourself with yourself in the past. That is you have to observe the changes in you that came after you started the journey from FAT TO FIT.

Keeping a track on your progress or on your journey will not just keep you motivated during the journey but it will also improve your analytical skills and thus improving your body along with your brain.

By observing yourself you will also be able to make the changes in your diet plan or workout plans if you did not progressed in your plans. It is same as the report cards that schools provide to the students after every month or twice so that they can keep a track on their progress and make changes in their study plan if progress in 0 or negative.

Tracking your progress will also make sure that are you on the right path or must be changing it! Some of the basic methods that I used to keep track on my journey are:

1. Observe your physical health. If you fell yourself active and energetic at your work or at home itself then it is a positive sign that signifies your positive progress. On contrary, I you fell exhausted and lazy then it's a sign of negative progress and you should rearrange your diet plan or workout plan.

2. You should observe your mental health as-well because along with physical fitness you should also have mental fitness. No doubt you might be physically getting transformed but your mental health might be not good. For example you are able to perform intense workouts properly but during the day you feel broke or unhappy with life, then these are signs that you are mentally unfit. To overcome this you have to check your diet plan because your diet may not be as healthy for your brain as it is for your body. Sometimes you also feel fatigue if you are dehydrated so keep up with water and have atleast 2.5 liters of water every-day.

3. The simplest way to track your progress is standing on weighing machine every week as to check your weekly progress and making a weekly report.

4. The most easiest and active way to measure or track your fitness is by writing the time you take every day to complete your workout on a paper or your note-taker and then comparing your time after a week or 10 days. If, the time is decreasing then it is a sign that you have progressed and thus you are on the right path. So, keep it up.

Now, as you know the importance of tracking and also some methods to track your progress, it is my humble request to never ever skip this step or never ignore this aspect of weight loss because this is the only tool that will keep you motivated on your path and make your journey purposeful.

Thus, keep a note and always have a purpose.

ASPECT 6: REWARDING YOURSELF
REWARD YOURSELF AFTER EACH MILESTONE.

Rewarding is a very important human psychology as it encourages them to continue to do whatever they are doing. It is a sign of appreciation to anybody who is working on something and an honor to receive the reward.

If you are a parent or you might have seen parents rewarding their child with a gift or a candy or anything that the child likes to have when the child have achieved good grades or he/she might have won any tournament of any sport. This is nothing but a 'keep it up' sign that will encourage the child to do even better and more in further life.

You might also know that schools provide scholarships to rankers and brilliant students as a note to keep it up with their studies and be better every-time. This will not just encourage the rankers but it will also inspire other students to study hard and get better grades so that they also get scholarship.

The sincere employees of any company are also rewarded with 'best employee award' and a bonus prize to just keep them doing their work without complaining and to inspire other employees to work hard to get that award and bonus.

Even in a match the best sports person is given a 'man of the match' award after the match to encourage them and to inspire other players to do their best in the next match.

In the above ways the people are rewarded to encourage them to do something good and keep it up, you also have to reward yourself with something you love to encourage yourself after you have achieved your milestone of weight loss.

Say for example, your goal is to lose 25 kg weight, then divide it into 5 milestones each of 5 kg. after working hard to lose weight when you reach the first 5 kg milestone then reward yourself with a piece of cake or a slice of your favorite pizza. This will encourage you to do more and keep you going on your path.

Thus it is a human tendency to keep going when rewarded for the work. Thus never forget to reward yourself when you achieve your milestones.

ASPECT 7: KNOWING A PATH AHEAD AFTER LOSING WEIGHT.

After you have successfully achieved your goal of losing weight there arises three options to fitness and it's your choice to choose a best one according to your will and need.

1. Maintain your body after losing weight: this is the most chosen option after losing weight as it is for common people like employees, bar-tenders and similar people doing normal job. As they don't need to further change their body they concentrate on maintaining their physique and just living a happy and normal life.

2. Muscle building (bulking up): if your goal is to do heavy-weight lifting or pursuing a career in sports then you can go for muscle building as it will help you best at your profession. You can also go for this if your dream is to have a muscular body or to just impress your girlfriend.

3. Shredding your body: if your goal is to become a model or pursue a career in film-industry or just a dream to become shredded then you can go for shredding your body. I am working on the same.

Once you have lose weight, never make a mistake of gaining that much weight back and always stay on the fit path.

I hope you loved the book and also suggest the book to them who you think can change their life.